Natural Medicine for Preppers

Your Guide to Using Plants, Herbs, and Essential Oils to Prepare for Any Emergency

MAIA HINES

All rights reserved. © 2023 by Maia Hines. No part of publication may be reproduced, distributed, or transmitted in any form or by any means, including photocopying, recording, or other electronic or mechanical methods, without the prior written permission of the publisher, except in the case of brief quotations embodied in critical reviews and certain other noncommercial uses permitted by copyright law.

Table of contents

INTRODUCTION

Welcome to Natural Medicine for Preppers

Natural Medicine for Preppers is a comprehensive guide designed to empower individuals with the knowledge and skills needed to integrate herbal remedies into their emergency preparedness plans. As our world faces various uncertainties and potential crises, the utilization of natural medicine becomes a crucial aspect of self-reliance. In this guide, we embark on a journey exploring the vast realm of herbal remedies, delving into the rich history, practical applications, and the intrinsic connection between nature and prepping.

The Importance of Herbal Remedies in Emergency Preparedness

In the face of unforeseen events, the reliance on traditional herbal remedies takes center stage as a fundamental component of emergency preparedness.

Understanding the historical significance of herbal medicine provides a solid foundation for preppers. Throughout centuries, diverse cultures have embraced the healing properties of plants, recognizing their efficacy in treating ailments and injuries. This chapter explores the timeless wisdom embedded in herbal practices, shedding light on the versatility and resilience that herbal remedies bring to the prepper's toolkit.

As preppers navigate the complexities of modern life, the significance of herbal remedies becomes even more pronounced. Unlike synthetic medications, herbal remedies often offer a holistic approach to health, addressing not only specific symptoms but also promoting overall well-being. This chapter delves into the diverse array of medicinal plants, emphasizing their role as a sustainable and natural alternative in times of crisis. By cultivating a deep understanding of these botanical allies, preppers can fortify their preparedness strategies with the timeless wisdom of herbal medicine.

Understanding Essential Oils and Their Role in Prepping

Essential oils, derived from aromatic plants, emerge as potent allies in the prepper's journey towards self-sufficiency. This chapter explores the extraction methods, properties, and versatile applications of essential oils in emergency preparedness. The distillation process, capturing the essence of plants, is unveiled as a meticulous art that transforms nature's aromatic gifts into concentrated therapeutic agents.

Essential oils go beyond their pleasant fragrances; they encapsulate the healing potential of plants in concentrated form. From lavender's calming properties to tea tree oil's antiseptic abilities, preppers can harness a diverse range of benefits. This chapter delves into the specific essential oils relevant to emergency situations, offering insights into creating blends for first aid, stress relief, and overall health maintenance. Understanding the nuances of essential oils enriches the prepper's toolkit, elevating their ability to address various challenges through the aromatic wisdom of nature.

Navigating Ahead

In the following chapters, we will embark on a journey through the foundations of natural medicine, building a herbal medicine cabinet, and integrating these powerful remedies into prepping plans for specific scenarios. This guide is not just about survival; it is about thriving in harmony with the abundant gifts nature provides, ensuring a resilient and holistic approach to emergency preparedness.

CHAPTER 1

Foundations of Natural Medicine

Historical Perspectives on Herbal Medicine

To truly appreciate the foundations of natural medicine, it is essential to delve into the historical tapestry of herbal medicine. Throughout the annals of time, diverse cultures across the globe have cultivated a profound relationship with medicinal plants. Ancient civilizations, such as the Egyptians, Greeks, and Chinese, embraced the healing properties of herbs, leaving behind a legacy that underscores the enduring efficacy of botanical remedies.

Herbal medicine has been intricately woven into the fabric of human existence, addressing a myriad of ailments and injuries long before the advent of modern pharmaceuticals. The knowledge passed down through generations reflects a deep understanding of the synergy between plants and the human body. In this historical exploration, we uncover the wisdom embedded in the practices of our ancestors, acknowledging the timeless relevance of herbal remedies in the context of emergency preparedness.

Basics of Botany: Identifying and Growing Medicinal Plants

The foundation of natural medicine rests upon a fundamental understanding of botany – the science of plants. Identifying and growing medicinal plants form the core of this knowledge base. Botanical literacy is paramount for preppers seeking self-reliance in times of crisis. In this section, we embark on a journey into the fascinating world of plant life, exploring the anatomy, taxonomy, and morphology of medicinal plants.

Learning to identify key plant species is a skill that transcends the theoretical; it is a practical necessity for those venturing into natural medicine. This chapter provides insights into recognizing medicinal plants in their natural habitats, understanding their growth patterns, and differentiating between beneficial herbs and potentially harmful look-alikes. Armed with this botanical acumen, preppers can confidently cultivate their herbal allies, fostering a symbiotic relationship with nature to enhance their emergency preparedness.

Sustainable Harvesting and Cultivation Practices

The sustainable cultivation and harvesting of medicinal plants lie at the heart of responsible herbalism. As stewards of the environment, preppers must be mindful of their impact on the delicate balance of ecosystems. This section explores ethical harvesting practices, emphasizing the importance of responsible gathering to ensure the longevity of medicinal plant populations.

Cultivating medicinal plants in a sustainable manner further solidifies the prepper's commitment to self-sufficiency. From creating herbal gardens to understanding permaculture principles, this chapter provides practical guidance on cultivating a renewable source of natural medicine. By embracing sustainable practices, preppers not only safeguard the environment but also ensure a continuous supply of medicinal herbs for their emergency preparedness endeavors.

CHAPTER 2

Building Your Herbal Medicine Cabinet

Essential Herbs for Preppers: A Comprehensive Guide

Building a robust herbal medicine cabinet is a cornerstone of effective prepping. This chapter embarks on a detailed exploration of essential herbs that preppers should include in their repertoire. Each herb carries a unique set of medicinal properties, making it a valuable asset in addressing a range of health concerns. From immune-boosting herbs like echinacea to versatile healing plants like aloe vera, this comprehensive guide equips preppers with the knowledge to select and cultivate the most relevant herbs for their needs.

The guide delves into the therapeutic actions of each herb, elucidating their historical uses and contemporary applications. Understanding the chemical constituents responsible for their healing properties enhances the prepper's ability to harness the full potential of these botanical allies. Whether it's the anti-inflammatory effects of turmeric or the soothing properties of chamomile, this chapter provides a nuanced understanding of how each herb contributes to a well-rounded herbal medicine cabinet.

Herbal Infusions, Decoctions, and Tinctures

Once the foundational herbs are identified, the next step in building a comprehensive herbal medicine cabinet is mastering the art of herbal preparations. Herbal infusions, decoctions, and tinctures emerge as essential techniques, each offering a unique method of extracting and preserving the medicinal properties of herbs.

Herbal infusions involve steeping herbs in hot water to extract their soluble compounds. This method is ideal for delicate herbs like peppermint or chamomile. Decoctions, on the other hand, involve simmering tougher plant parts, such as roots or bark, to extract their therapeutic components. Understanding the subtleties between these methods allows preppers to tailor their preparations to the specific needs of each herb.

Tinctures, alcohol-based extracts, offer a concentrated and long-lasting form of herbal medicine. This chapter guides preppers through the process of creating tinctures, exploring the appropriate alcohol percentages and ratios for optimal extraction. By mastering these techniques, preppers not only ensure the potency of their herbal medicines but also enhance their ability to store and administer remedies effectively.

Creating Your First Aid Herbal Kit

A first aid herbal kit is a vital component of any prepper's emergency preparedness strategy. This section guides preppers in assembling a well-rounded herbal first aid kit, incorporating the essential herbs and preparations covered earlier. From cuts and bruises to digestive issues and respiratory ailments, the first aid kit becomes a versatile resource for addressing a spectrum of health concerns in emergency situations.

The chapter outlines the specific herbs and herbal preparations suitable for inclusion in the first aid kit. Practical considerations, such as storage and shelf life, are explored to ensure the longevity and efficacy of the herbal remedies. By creating a personalized first aid herbal kit, preppers not only enhance their ability to address health emergencies but also foster a deeper connection with the natural world and its healing offerings.

Navigating Ahead

In the subsequent chapters, we will explore the integration of natural medicine into prepping plans, focusing on incorporating herbal remedies into emergency food supplies and enhancing everyday preparedness with the power of herbal solutions. As preppers build their herbal medicine knowledge and practical skills, they construct a resilient foundation for self-sufficiency in times of need.

CHAPTER 3

Harnessing the Power of Essential Oils

Introduction to Essential Oils and Their Extraction Methods

Essential oils, the concentrated aromatic compounds derived from plants, stand as potent allies in the realm of natural medicine. This chapter initiates a comprehensive exploration by providing an introduction to essential oils and elucidating the intricate process of their extraction. The art of distillation, steam distillation being the most common method, is unveiled as a meticulous process that captures the essence of aromatic plants, producing highly concentrated and therapeutic oils.

The discussion extends to the varied extraction methods, including cold pressing and solvent extraction, each imparting distinct characteristics to the final product. Understanding the intricacies of these methods empowers preppers to make informed choices when selecting and utilizing essential oils. As preppers delve into the world of aromatics, they gain insights into the alchemy that transforms botanical substances into concentrated remedies, ready to address a myriad of health concerns.

Essential Oils for Common Ailments and Injuries

Essential oils, with their diverse therapeutic properties, offer preppers a natural and versatile toolkit for addressing common ailments and injuries. This section delves into the specific essential oils relevant to emergency situations, providing a comprehensive guide for preppers. From lavender's calming effects to tea tree oil's antiseptic properties, essential oils become invaluable resources in the prepper's journey towards self-reliance.

The chapter explores the application of essential oils in managing respiratory issues, alleviating pain, and promoting overall well-being. Whether combating headaches, soothing insect bites, or supporting the immune system, the curated selection of essential oils becomes a holistic approach to health maintenance. By understanding the nuanced benefits of each oil, preppers can strategically incorporate them into their emergency preparedness plans, fostering resilience in the face of health challenges.

Blending Essential Oils for Maximum Effectiveness

While individual essential oils carry potent therapeutic properties, blending them strategically enhances their effectiveness. This section guides preppers through the art of blending essential oils, considering factors such as synergy, aroma, and intended therapeutic outcomes. From creating custom blends for stress relief to formulating potent antiviral combinations, the prepper becomes an artisan in crafting aromatic solutions tailored to their specific needs.

Navigating Ahead

The chapter explores the concept of base, middle, and top notes in blending, allowing preppers to create well-balanced and harmonious aromatic compositions. Safety considerations, such as dilution ratios and potential contraindications, are also addressed to ensure responsible and effective usage. As preppers delve into the realm of blending, they unlock the full potential of essential oils, transforming them into personalized remedies that resonate with their individual health goals.

In the subsequent chapters, we will integrate natural medicine into prepping plans, exploring the incorporation of herbal remedies into emergency food supplies and infusing bug-out bags with the power of herbal solutions. As preppers harness the power of essential oils, they add another layer to their holistic approach to emergency preparedness, where aromatic remedies become a fragrant and potent arsenal in times of need.

CHAPTER 4

Integrating Natural Medicine into Prepping Plans

Incorporating Herbal Remedies into Emergency Food Supplies

The integration of natural medicine into prepping plans requires a strategic approach, and one pivotal aspect is incorporating herbal remedies into emergency food supplies. This chapter explores the synergy between nutrition and herbalism, providing preppers with insights into fortifying their sustenance with medicinal plants. From dehydrated herbs for seasoning to powdered herbs for nutritional enhancement, the possibilities are diverse and can significantly contribute to overall well-being during times of crisis.

The chapter navigates through the essential herbs that complement emergency food supplies. These herbs not only add flavor and nutritional value but also bring a medicinal dimension to the prepper's sustenance strategy. Considerations such as shelf stability, ease of preparation, and compatibility with various food items are addressed, ensuring that herbal remedies seamlessly integrate into the prepper's long-term emergency provisions.

Herbal First Aid: Strategies for Prepping and Survival

First aid is a cornerstone of emergency preparedness, and integrating herbal remedies into this paradigm enhances the prepper's ability to address health issues effectively. This section delves into herbal first aid strategies, providing a comprehensive guide for preppers to navigate injuries and illnesses in austere environments. From cuts and burns to respiratory distress and digestive discomfort, herbal first aid becomes a versatile and holistic approach to health management.

The chapter outlines specific herbs and their applications in first aid scenarios, emphasizing the importance of a well-rounded herbal first aid kit. Practical considerations, such as storage conditions and accessibility, are explored to ensure that preppers can deploy their herbal remedies swiftly and efficiently when needed. By understanding the principles of herbal first aid, preppers not only enhance their medical preparedness but also cultivate a deeper connection with the healing properties of nature.

Natural Medicine in Bug Out Bags and Everyday Preparedness

Bug-out bags are essential components of prepping for various scenarios, and integrating natural medicine into these kits adds a layer of resilience. This section explores the strategic inclusion of herbal solutions in bug-out bags, ensuring that preppers have access to vital remedies during evacuation or survival scenarios. Lightweight and versatile herbal preparations, such as tinctures and herbal salves, become invaluable assets in the prepper's mobile medical kit.

The chapter extends beyond bug-out bags to everyday preparedness, emphasizing the integration of herbal remedies into daily routines. From herbal teas for stress relief to salves for minor injuries, natural medicine becomes a seamless and integral part of the prepper's lifestyle. By adopting a proactive approach to health maintenance, preppers cultivate resilience and self-sufficiency, minimizing the reliance on conventional medical resources in times of need.

Navigating Ahead

In the subsequent chapters, we will delve into specific scenarios, exploring herbal solutions for respiratory issues, digestive health, and stress management. As preppers navigate the integration of natural medicine into their preparedness plans, they weave a comprehensive strategy where herbs are not just supplements but essential components of a resilient and holistic approach to health and survival.

CHAPTER 5

Prepping for Specific Scenarios

Herbal Solutions for Respiratory Issues

Respiratory issues can pose significant challenges in emergency scenarios, and this chapter explores the herbal solutions available for preppers to address such concerns. From common colds to more severe respiratory infections, a range of medicinal plants offers relief and support. Herbs like eucalyptus, thyme, and peppermint, known for their expectorant and decongestant properties, become essential components of the prepper's toolkit.

The chapter provides detailed insights into creating herbal steam inhalations, teas, and tinctures specifically tailored for respiratory health. Understanding the mechanisms through which these herbs work – whether by soothing irritated airways or promoting mucus clearance – empowers preppers to make informed choices in managing respiratory issues effectively. By integrating herbal solutions into their preparedness plans, preppers fortify their respiratory health and enhance their resilience against airborne threats.

Natural Remedies for Digestive Health

Maintaining digestive health is crucial for overall well-being, and in the context of emergency preparedness, it becomes paramount. This section explores natural remedies for digestive health, focusing on herbs that address common gastrointestinal issues. From soothing herbs like chamomile and ginger to digestive bitters such as gentian, preppers can create a diverse array of herbal preparations to support optimal digestive function.

The chapter delves into the art of crafting herbal teas, infusions, and tinctures that aid digestion, alleviate indigestion, and promote gut health. The role of probiotic-rich herbs in fostering a balanced gut microbiome is also highlighted, emphasizing the interconnectedness of digestive health with the broader immune system. As preppers navigate the integration of herbal remedies for digestive well-being, they not only ensure their physical resilience but also cultivate a holistic approach to health in the face of uncertainty.

Herbal Approaches to Stress, Anxiety, and Sleep Disorders

Stress, anxiety, and sleep disorders can significantly impact an individual's ability to navigate challenging scenarios. This section explores herbal approaches to promoting mental well-being and managing stress-related challenges. Adaptogenic herbs like ashwagandha and rhodiola, known for their ability to modulate the body's stress response, become crucial allies for preppers seeking emotional resilience.

The chapter delves into the calming properties of herbs such as valerian, passionflower, and lemon balm, offering natural alternatives to address anxiety and promote restful sleep. The nuanced art of herbal formulation for stress management is explored, guiding preppers in creating blends that resonate with their individual needs. By integrating herbal approaches to mental health into their preparedness plans, preppers foster emotional strength and equip themselves to face uncertainties with a centered and resilient mindset.

Navigating Ahead

In the subsequent chapters, we will further explore
the practical applications of natural medicine,
examining ways to integrate herbal cleaning
products, eco-friendly pest control, and herbal
beauty and personal care into everyday prepping. As
preppers tailor their strategies for specific scenarios,
they intricately weave herbal remedies into the
fabric of their preparedness, creating a resilient
foundation for holistic health and survival.

CHAPTER 6

Home Remedies for Sustainable Living

Herbal Cleaning Products and Natural Disinfectants

The integration of natural medicine extends beyond health remedies to encompass sustainable living practices within the home. This chapter explores the realm of herbal cleaning products and natural disinfectants, providing preppers with eco-friendly alternatives to conventional household cleaners. From citrus-infused vinegar solutions to herbal antimicrobial blends, preppers can craft cleaning products that are not only effective but also environmentally conscious.

The chapter delves into the antimicrobial properties of herbs such as tea tree, thyme, and lavender, showcasing their potential as natural disinfectants. Understanding the synergy between herbs and essential oils in creating potent cleaning solutions empowers preppers to maintain a clean and hygienic living environment without resorting to harsh chemicals. By incorporating herbal cleaning products into their sustainable living practices, preppers contribute to a healthier home and planet.

Eco-Friendly Pest Control Using Plants

Pest control often involves the use of synthetic chemicals that can have adverse effects on the environment. In this section, preppers are introduced to the concept of eco-friendly pest control using plants. Certain herbs possess natural insect-repelling properties, making them effective allies in managing pests without compromising environmental sustainability. Plants like citronella, peppermint, and neem become botanical guardians, deterring insects from invading homes and gardens.

The chapter explores various methods of incorporating these pest-repelling plants into daily life, from planting them strategically in gardens to creating herbal repellent sprays. Understanding the lifecycle of common pests and the specific plants that disrupt their breeding and feeding patterns empowers preppers to take a proactive and natural approach to pest control. By embracing eco-friendly pest control using plants, preppers not only safeguard their living spaces but also contribute to the broader goal of sustainable and harmonious coexistence with nature.

Herbal Beauty and Personal Care Prepping

Sustainable living encompasses more than just the environment; it extends to personal care practices that prioritize natural ingredients and reduce reliance on commercial products laden with synthetic chemicals. This section explores herbal beauty and personal care prepping, inviting preppers to craft their own skincare and hygiene products using botanical ingredients.

The chapter delves into the properties of herbs like aloe vera, calendula, and chamomile, highlighting their skin-soothing and nourishing attributes. Preppers can learn to create herbal-infused oils, balms, and salves that cater to individual skincare needs. Beyond skincare, herbal solutions for natural deodorants, toothpaste, and hair care are explored, offering preppers a diverse toolkit for maintaining personal hygiene without compromising on sustainability.

As preppers embrace herbal beauty and personal care prepping, they not only reduce their environmental footprint but also gain a deeper connection with the healing potential of nature. By cultivating a self-sufficient and sustainable approach to personal care, preppers contribute to a broader ethos of mindful living, where herbal remedies extend seamlessly into every aspect of their daily routines.

Navigating Ahead

In the subsequent chapters, we will conclude our journey through the comprehensive guide to natural medicine for preppers. We will revisit key principles, reinforce practical applications, and emphasize the overarching theme of resilience and self-sufficiency that herbal remedies bring to the prepper's lifestyle. As we navigate the final chapters, the integration of natural medicine into prepping plans becomes a holistic and sustainable endeavor, creating a resilient foundation for thriving in harmony with the natural world.

CONCLUSION

Embracing the Power of Natural Medicine in Preparedness

The journey through the comprehensive guide to natural medicine for preppers culminates in the profound realization of the transformative power inherent in herbal remedies. Embracing the power of natural medicine in preparedness extends beyond the acquisition of knowledge; it becomes a philosophy, a way of life that intertwines resilience, self-sufficiency, and a harmonious relationship with the natural world. Through the exploration of historical perspectives, the fundamentals of botany, and the integration of herbal solutions into various aspects of life, preppers embark on a holistic journey towards wellness and preparedness.

The essence of natural medicine lies in its ability to forge a connection between humanity and the abundant gifts of nature. Herbal remedies, extracted from the very plants that have sustained civilizations for centuries, offer a timeless and sustainable approach to health and well-being. As preppers delve into the intricacies of herbal preparations, from infusions and tinctures to herbal first aid kits and eco-friendly pest control, they discover a rich tapestry of knowledge that empowers them to navigate uncertainties with confidence.

The importance of herbal remedies in emergency preparedness cannot be overstated. From addressing common ailments to providing solutions for specific scenarios such as respiratory issues, digestive health, and mental well-being, natural medicine emerges as a versatile and effective toolkit for preppers. The chapters exploring essential herbs, the power of essential oils, and the integration of herbal solutions into prepping plans lay the foundation for a resilient and comprehensive approach to preparedness.

The embrace of natural medicine goes beyond the individual; it extends to sustainable living practices within the home. Herbal cleaning products, natural disinfectants, and eco-friendly pest control become integral components of a prepper's lifestyle, fostering a commitment to environmental consciousness. Through the creation of herbal beauty and personal care products, preppers not only prioritize self-sufficiency but also contribute to a culture of mindful living that respects and honors the delicate balance of nature.

As preppers navigate their journey in herbal prepping, they become stewards of their health, guardians of their homes, and champions of sustainability. The potency of herbal remedies lies not only in their medicinal properties but also in their ability to cultivate a deeper connection with the natural world. This connection, forged through the careful cultivation of medicinal plants, the crafting of herbal remedies, and the incorporation of natural medicine into daily life, transforms prepping from a practical necessity into a holistic and fulfilling lifestyle.

Moving Forward: Your Journey in Herbal Prepping

The conclusion of this guide marks the beginning of a personal journey for every prepper committed to herbal remedies and self-sufficiency. Moving forward, the journey in herbal prepping is an ongoing exploration, a continuous learning process that adapts to individual needs, circumstances, and the evolving landscape of health and preparedness. Here are key aspects to consider as you embark on your unique path in herbal prepping:

Cultivate a Relationship with Medicinal Plants

As you move forward, deepen your connection with medicinal plants. Consider creating a dedicated space for growing herbs or participating in local initiatives that promote sustainable gardening. By cultivating a relationship with these botanical allies, you not only secure a renewable source of herbal remedies but also foster a sense of reciprocity with the natural world.

Expand Your Herbal Toolkit

The world of herbal medicine is vast, and there is always more to discover. Explore new herbs, experiment with different preparations, and expand your herbal toolkit. Attend workshops, connect with herbalists, and engage with the vibrant community of individuals passionate about natural medicine. By continuously broadening your knowledge, you enrich your ability to address a variety of health concerns.

Integrate Natural Medicine into Daily Life

Herbal prepping is not reserved solely for emergencies; it is a way of life. Integrate natural medicine into your daily routines, from herbal teas in the morning to herbal-infused skincare in the evening. By incorporating herbal remedies into everyday life, you fortify your well-being and establish a sustainable approach to health.

Share Your Knowledge

As you accumulate knowledge and experience in herbal prepping, consider sharing your insights with others. Whether within your community, through online platforms, or by hosting workshops, sharing your knowledge contributes to a collective understanding of natural medicine. This exchange of wisdom fosters a supportive network of individuals committed to self-sufficiency and herbal wellness.

Adapt to Changing Circumstances

The landscape of preparedness is dynamic, and adaptability is a key attribute for any prepper. As you move forward in your herbal prepping journey, remain open to adapting your strategies based on changing circumstances. Explore new herbal solutions, reassess your emergency plans, and refine your approach to align with evolving needs.

In conclusion, the journey in herbal prepping is a tapestry of learning, discovery, and resilience. By embracing the power of natural medicine, preppers not only equip themselves for emergencies but also cultivate a lifestyle that harmonizes with the inherent wisdom of the natural world. As you move forward on this path, may your herbal preparations be a source of empowerment, your knowledge a beacon of self-sufficiency, and your journey a testament to the transformative potential of herbal remedies in preparedness.

www.ingramcontent.com/pod-product-compliance
Lightning Source LLC
Chambersburg PA
CBHW070751260726

48660CB00007B/3065